A Comprehensive Yoga Guide

Learn Yogic Postures For Stress Relief, Weight Loss, And Meditation

By

Meenakshi Narang

Table of Contents

INTRODUCTION

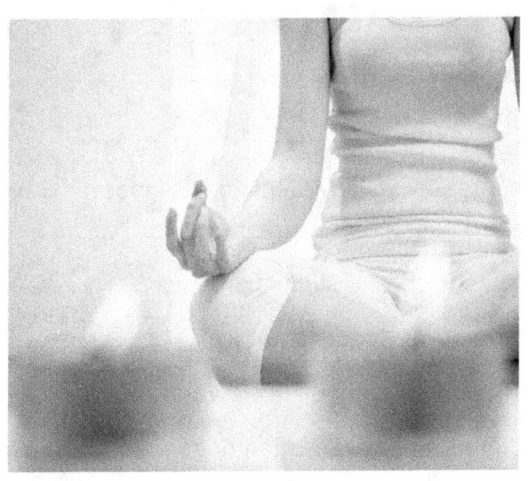

Human life needs comprehensive conditioning for its holistic growth. Whilst, modern times lay stress on artificial modes of gratification and conditioning, the truest healing and nurturing will come only from natural methods, one is Yoga. Yoga is no longer new to many of us. However, a correct and simplified interpretation of Yoga is always desirable so that it would bring more understanding on this meta-physical discipline. This book is one such effort to bring the fundamentals of Yoga right into our palms. You will learn about its various postures and their benefits.

This comprehensive Yoga guide will render answers to all the queries that you might have. This book is an attempt to bring in the basics of Yoga to make our lives better and healthier. The easy-to-understand descriptions of various postures and Yogic kriyas (procedures) will certainly help readers in understanding Yoga and getting the most of its Health benefits.

Happy Reading!

Chapter 1 - Yoga For Amateurs

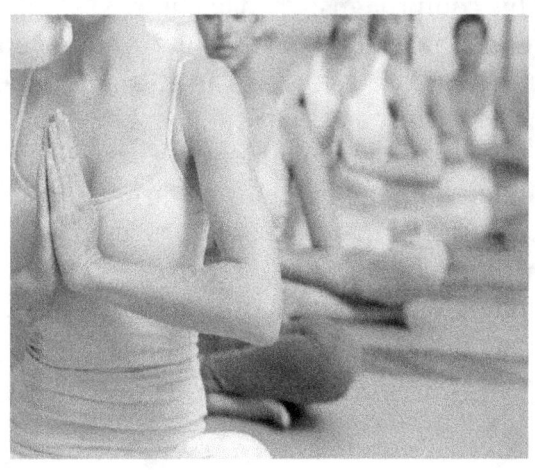

What is Yoga

Yoga is the earliest form of physical discipline recorded in human life on earth. The exact origin of yoga is debatable however it is thought to be around fifty centuries old. The earliest known sighting of yoga according to experts traces back to around 3000 B.C. The intention of several yoga postures and exercises was to enhance mental strength and give relaxation to the practitioners without tiring them, so as to prepare for rigorous meditation while being alert for long periods of time.

Yoga is a science that helps an individual search for their soul and establishes unity between the individual of finite existence and the infinite divine spiritual force. Yoga is a concept where the body is connected to the breath; both are interconnected to the brain; in turn these link with the mind, which forms our mental ability of consciousness.

Yoga is a form of exercise of the body and mind that is based on upon the intimate connection between the body, breathing, and mind. By manipulation of breath and stabilizing the body in postures called asanas, yoga achieves harmony. Through yoga, an individual can balance and regulate their body, mind, and in-depth feelings to withdraw themselves from the chaos of the world and find inner peace.

Yoga achieves this by using movement, breath, stability, relaxation and meditation to construct a healthy, stable and a positive approach to life.

The real purpose of yoga is to gain control of your life by controlling three factors, the body, breath, and mind. Control and balance are what an individual could benefit from while practicing yoga, apart from other advantages. In every aspect of life, yoga represents balanced moderation.

Yoga in Modern Life

The system of yoga followed now in western countries is called Hatha yoga. Hatha Yoga is the union between two separate entities, interdependent but separate. This is suggestive of the healthy collaboration of extremes - in this case, the mind and body - which leads to strength, vitality and a feeling of satisfaction.

Hatha yoga is strongly based upon the practice of postures, various breathing techniques (called pranayama) and meditation for overall development. It aims to regulate the flow of energy in and out of the body as a form of exercise. The asanas or postures emphasize with controlled movement, focus, flexibility, and deep breathing. There are nearly 200 asanas of which more than half are practiced widely in the world. The asana postures vary from very simple to a complex that can be easily achieved and extremely challenging respectively. Even though, the movements are slower and controlled; Hatha Yoga provides the individual with a complete and thorough workout for the mind and body.

Yoga is not a Religion

Although yoga is associated with spirituality, it is not the ideal definition of a religion. Rather than broadcasting a philosophy, hatha yoga is a physical and psychological discipline that integrates the learning and practice of asanas, pranayama, and meditation together.

The yoga principles include five yamas that follow paths of non-violence; truthfulness; honesty; chastity; and generosity. There is another set of five principles called niyamas that symbolize purity; contentment; self-discipline; self-study; and divine spirituality.

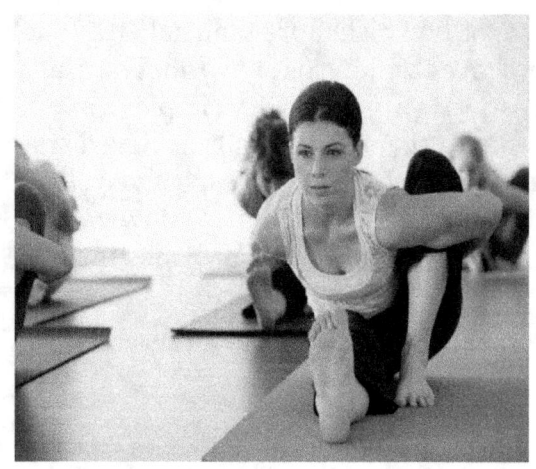

Get Committed to Yoga

The first step, to getting committed to yoga, is to make sure that you want to practice yoga. To analyze your requirement of practicing yoga you need to take that next step and start enjoying the relaxation and benefits of yoga.

1. Decide Kind of Yoga

Although there are many yoga classes out there, choosing the right one is extremely important as picking one that doesn't match your physical build type could seem irritating. Often for beginners, a Hatha or Vinyasa class is considered ideal, varying with speed, as a slow or fast-paced class. These are basic and primary types, with several other fancier types and exercises.

2. Locate Yoga Class

Find a class that is equidistant from your workplace and home so as to make it convenient to get to your home or work easily. Start with a beginner level class that you can find in several gyms. Find a good teacher for your initial classes and keep trying until you find one you like. You can find a yoga class in your area of residence through several websites. For further information, you can also look at local newspapers or health magazines for listings and advertisements.

3. Carry your enthusiasm

As you progress with extreme exercises, read up on basic yoga equipment you will require like yoga mats. Yoga isn't often associated with equipment. It's one of a kind that requires only the presence of the individual.

In a typical yoga class setting, the students place their mats facing their teacher's mat in a loose matrix formation. It indicates the front of the room and is often identifiable by a small altar. Leave some space between you and your neighbor's mat as you will need to stretch your arms and body for certain exercises and postures. The students often sit in a cross-legged position and warm up their bodies before any serious exercises.

The teacher initiates the class by chanting the word "OM" three times. This chanting is a form of warm up as the vibration is felt all over the body. This is followed with a breathing exercise or short meditation. Warm-up postures follow with the complexity increasing gradually and then followed up by relaxation. Most teachers end class with another chanting round of OM to calm the body down.

After the first day or class, you may feel a little sore at the end of the day.

What To DO And What NOT TO

- Heavy meal should not be consumed before practicing yoga. Before class hours, eat light
- Don't drink water during the exercises. Have it either before or after
- Don't wear shoes or socks while practicing Yoga
- Do take tips on yoga from the internet on how to improve yourself
- Do review case studies of yoga experts, so you take lesser time to adapt
- Do inform the trainer if it's your first class, the extra attention would be helpful.
- Do ask for help whenever required
- Do familiarize with the terminology so you don't feel out of place.

Chapter 2 – Yogic Postures For Shedding Excess Weight

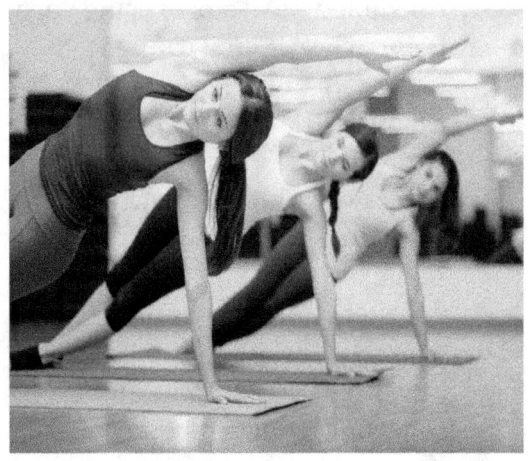

Many aspirants practice yoga to get in control of their body and ultimately shed kilos of their body to get a perfect and lean figure. You will have to perfect few of the postures of yoga to lose weight. Weight loss through yoga isn't a one-week affair and takes several months of training and regular yoga.

Many people experiment with several different things to get into perfect shape. Only exercises and workouts will accumulate the body strength by toning down the muscles, thereby losing on fat.

The following postures help you in flattening your stomach.

Warrior Posture:

Raise your hands above your head and stretch them as long as possible. Clasp your hands together to make a Namaste gesture and turn yourself to the right. Bend your right knee a little while trying to stretch your abdominal muscles as much as possible. Repeat the procedure on the left side. This is beneficial as it tightens your muscles and reduces fat deposited in the legs giving you an impressive body built.

Warrior Posture II:

This yoga posture focuses on another kind of muscles and is just as important. It has the same effect on the tummy and legs. It is done in a unique way. The hands do not make a Namaste gesture rather they are stretched out to both the sides while the leg is bent. This has advantages as this posture stretches abdominal muscles for effective fat elimination.

Chair Posture:

With this asana, you will experience pain in your legs for the initial couple of days. As you practice it, the pain eases out. You will have to keep your feet together. Inhale as you raise your hands above head level. Stretch them up and bend your knees slightly, make sure keep inhaling while bending. Now the difficult part, hold this position for at least 60 seconds. It will make sure you have toned thighs and melt your tummy fat.

Boat Posture:

Sit down on your yoga mat and stretch your legs out. Your knees should be pulled up, thighs should be kept tight and toes pointed out. Now gradually raise your feet off the ground and set them at a 45-degree angle. Keep inhaling as you raise your feet and try not to bend your knees. Keep your spine erect.

Bridge Posture:

Lie straight down on your back and bend your knees, make sure your feet are firmly on the ground. Place hands on the ground and keep them straight. Raise your hips from the ground and try to balance your body. This posture will improve your muscle strength and efficiency. You can also experiment by adding variations to this posture. Lift one leg in the air for longer periods of time.

Cobbler posture:

Cobbler posture is one of the most simplest and advantageous postures of yoga. Sit down with your spine erect. Your knees should be bent and the soles of your feet facing each other. Press your soles together and hold this posture for a minute.

Locust Posture:

Lie face down while your palms face the ground. Inhale a burst of fresh air while lifting up your legs without bending your knees. The upper side of your stomach and hands should also be lifted to stretch your abdominal muscles. This posture helps you to minimize the fat zones near the hips and expand the ability of leg muscles.

Camel Posture:

Sit on your feet with your knees and calves very close. You will have to place a soft cloth under to prevent pain. After doing so, come onto your knees and place your hands on your hips while stretching out the torso. Hold your heels gradually one after the other and try to bend backward to expand your chest and tummy. Try feeling the weight of your body in your arms. This posture is very beneficial to reduce accumulated fat in the whole body.

This will burn most of your fats and give you a healthier, regularly-shaped body. They also help you to lose unhealthy fat accumulation in the body tissues.

Moreover, conditions like constipation, stress and hypersensitivity are significantly reduced by these postures. Through these yoga postures designed for weight loss, you can develop a sound mind and an even better body.

Chapter 3 - Yoga as Stress Buster

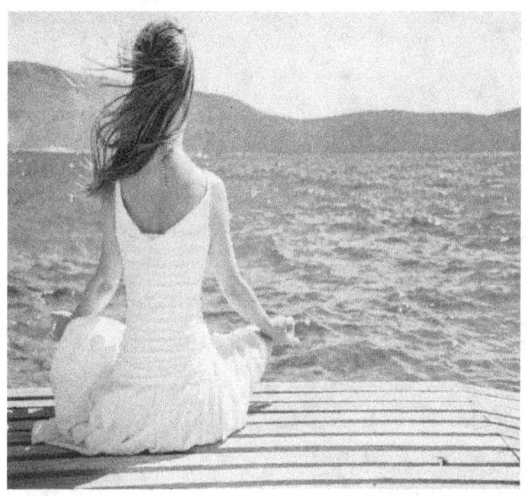

We all lead a very busy and stressful lives. Right from morning till evening, we are struggling to make our ends meet. We keep our minds as well as bodies indulged in various activities that consciously / unconsciously take a toll on our peace of mind.

Apart from these, everyday issues can cause us emotional stress also — it could be counseling a friend going through tough times, regretting some argument with sibling, making up mind about a crucial decision, or thinking hard about the future. No doubt, it's usual to feel stressed.

Yoga for Relieving Stress

There are many ways that would alleviate stress from our lives including heart-to-heat communication and working out. Yoga promotes relaxation and reduces stress levels. It can improve on three aspects of our lives - our mind, body and breathing. One shouldn't feel stressed out to practice yoga, as it is an exercise to relieve stress rather than build it up. Those who practice yoga regularly tend to be calmer intense situations and show better response when things go out of hand. Practicing yoga amplifies your ability to calm, focus, balance, and relax yourself.

Practicing Comprehensive Yoga

Easier postures like the mountain posture are a stress reliever when you focus on keeping your breathing regulated and balanced, visualizing yourself as tough and steady as a mountain. When you're in a typical yoga posture, focus your mind on the harmony of your organs and how to unite your body, mind, and breathing.

Avoid Mental Wandering

Think about what your body and breath are doing in this moment. You will notice how every particular muscle or area of the body feels and responds. Focus on breathing slowly to make sure your body stretches tall while breathing out a burst of air as you curl up. When under pressure, we often find ourselves thinking about what we need to accomplish in the future or what we should have done better in the past. Instead of honoring the present by not letting your thoughts wander as you do yoga.

Living in the moment like this assists you in building your mental ability to focus and concentrate, which helps in every aspect of life. When the going gets tough, utilize your breathing. When a particular yoga posture seems challenging, send your breath to the area in your body which feels stiff or tight while practicing. This skill can be applied in various scenarios for the rest of your life. Whenever something in your daily routine challenges you — a tough problem, regretting over a parent's decision — regulate your breathing. This simple solution will surprise you.

Practicing Yoga at the right time

Try taking weekly class and if daily not possible, purchase yoga DVD to help you learn and guide you through yoga postures. There are yoga classes and DVDs exclusively for students. You can also practice small tips regarding your trip in into your daily lift so as to help you stay calm in stressful moments.

Exercising before Exam

Do easy and simple neck and shoulder rolls right at your desk to relieve the muscles in your neck, shoulders, and back while trying to squeeze and relaxing your fingers and hands. These exercises can happen in smaller periods of time and repeated whenever you need.

At the time of studying

Neck and shoulder rolls can relieve the tension in your back and shoulders.

Forward folds and twists will release lower back strain levels. You can also give your face a small massage just to help loosen up a rigid jaw. Try a few easy yoga moves that help relaxing areas that may have been exposed to external stress or may have become tense while studying. Balancing postures, like the tree posture, can help focus our energy for you to use it for concentrating better on what you need to do.

Before sleeping

Yoga postures, where you fold forward, like a child, are said to be calming. They provide you with a chance to shut out the rest of the world and remain quiet and peaceful. Remain in a forward fold for few minutes and allow your body & mind to remain free from tension.

Chapter 4 – Staying Calm and Composed with Yogic Kriyas and Postures

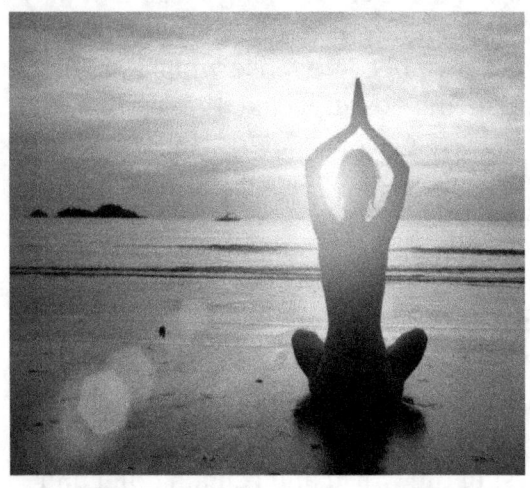

The Sudarshan Kriya is a 20-minute yoga/meditation exercise that involves integrated breathing techniques. This breathing exercise has a major effect on your body as it's widely known for its promising ability to eliminate stress and help a person focus entirely on the task at hand. In this, the main importance is given to the breathing patterns, something that is the most crucial aspect of life. Kriya helps in syncing your body, soul and mind. Inner peace can be achieved thereby releasing all the negative toxins from the body. Sudarshan Kriya is an exercise that enhances the physical, mental, emotional and social well-being of an individual and is an integral part of many yoga programs. It has influenced millions of lives and taught them how to celebrate life! Hence, it is important for one to learn and practice SudarshanKriya yoga for your spiritual, emotional and physical strength.

Significance of Sudarshan Kriya

Just like a daily morning bath, practicing Sudarshan Kriya daily is an important step as it cleanses 90% of our body internally. It eliminates excess stress, anxiety, depression and other factors that take a toll on the system. According to experts, a scientific experiment concluded that 20 minutes of Kriya equals 8 hours of effective sleep.

Practicing Sudarshan Kriya

Practicing SudarshanKriya Yoga regularly enhances the overall personality of a person. The technique though complicated can be done in four easy steps.

Follow these four steps:

Pranayama: The three stages are done while the individual is focused and is sitting in a Vajrasan posture (sitting with legs folded and ankle in contact with the hips). It comprises of 3 different and unique postures.

Bhastrika: Also followed under vajrasan in three sets with powerful and forceful breathing from the nose. After Bhastrika, the sitting posture shifts from vajrasan to sukhasan.

OM Chanting: This is to record the vibrations which have a positive effect on the body.

Three levels of breathing (slow, medium and fast)

Advantages of Practicing Vajrasan:

The sitting posture Vajrasan is also called by several other names based such as, Adamantine Posture Diamond Posture, Pelvic Posture, Kneeling Posture, and Thunderbolt Posture. The posture has a very significant role to play in effective yoga meditation. There are several benefits associated with vajrasan like:

- Tones the thigh muscles
- Better concentration levels
- Mental stability
- Cures digestive problems
- Cures stomach disorders
- Cures problematic conditions related to urine
- Natural back pain killer
- Amplifies blood circulation
- Minimize/Restrict obesity
- Acts as painkiller for arthritis patients

Importance of OM chanting

Chanting OM is very effective and beneficial as it improvises on the positive effect of Brahma, Vishnu and Shiva energy in the body. Brahma in Hindu mythology is the creator i.e it betters our creativity skills like writing, drawing and other skills. Vishnu means one who continues and does not give up i.e excellent management skills like volunteers, event coordinators. Shiva, the last principle, means destroyer i.e dynamic professions like doctor, engineer, etc.

Accumulation of negative toxins has become a large part helping in patterns of our lives like high-stress levels, anxiety, tension and many more. These qualities when in a proper association, can lead to diseases such cardiovascular ailments, asthma, HIV, and cancer, is able to make life worse. Therefore, it's very important to have some peace of mind which can be attained by practicing this yoga daily. It gives you immaculate mental abilities to deal with all problems while maintaining good health. It also betters your thinking capability, clarity of speech and feel harmonic and in accordance. Although, it is not an easy technique there have to several trial counts to spread the energy to the companion chain for everyone.

Regular Kriya practitioners have reported amplified immunity, increased stamina and sustained high-energy levels. It will also help you understand complex emotions like happiness, anger and sadness effectively.

Moreover, Sudarshan Kriya Yoga exercise does not have any particular side effects as it can be taught from both ends while keeping the effect on the body constant.

This is becoming so popular and it is important that you start practicing too. ⁇

Chapter 5 - Yogic Chakras

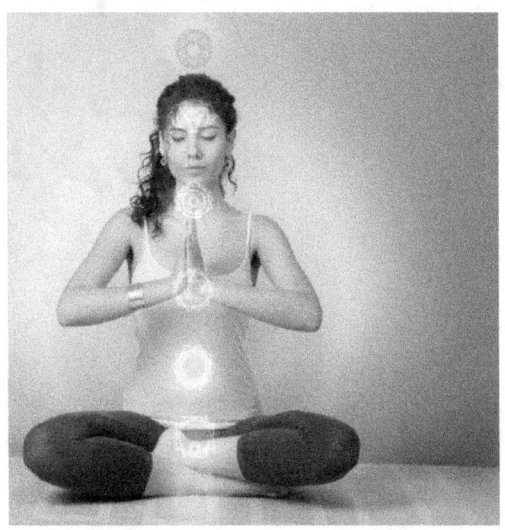

The Tantrik yogis who were experts in yoga meditation understood for an individual to honor a different kind of life—one with more stability, more peace, and better empathy levels— one has to change from within himself. Feel with inner power how energetic centers known as the yogic chakras work in accordance.

What does Yogic Chakras mean?

Chakra is a word derived from Sanskrit transcript and means "spinning wheel." As per yogic science, chakras are the convergence of energy, emotions, and the physical body. The point where our conscience and consciousness are projected together through these chakras which majorly determines how we live in the reality through our emotional reactions, our needs and weaknesses, our level of confidence or fear.

By understanding these centers in yoga meditation practice, we can take the first initial step to break down any blockades that would avoid us exploring our full potential.

Chakras

Root Chakra (Muladhara) - This yogic chakra center is located on the pelvic floor. It functions like a root, connecting us to the Earth. It keeps you grounded in the present reality while maintaining your physical strength and security. It holds your immature desires around food, sleep, sex, and survival. It regulates your opportunities and fears. Muladhara (Kundalini Shakti) controls our most powerful inner potential. Through yogic meditation, we give life to the internal inactive power that presides in our root. Various asanas such as Warrior stances, hip-openers, Chair Posture, deep lunges, and squats help in bringing attention to this center.

Svadishthana (Pelvic Chakra) - When our mind fluctuates uncontrollably through this area, we access our inner potential for self-healing and sensual pleasure. When this chakra is inactive to our consciousness, we become ruled by our needs and desires. Just like the root chakra, asanas like forward bending, squats and hip-openings help us bring awareness to this chakra. This yogic chakra resides in sacrum. It is the home of the reproductive organs and focal of our inherent desires.

Manipura(Navel Chakra) - The navel chakra is associated with the digestive system, also known as the element of fire, and individual abilities and desires. When our consciousness lies in this chakra, we become empowered by the energy of transformation whereas when it is blocked, we are uncontrollable and an imbalance occurs linked to aggressiveness, egoism, and the tyranny. Twists are the asanas that can heal and achieve manipura.

Anahata(Heart Chakra) - Right at the center of the chest, the heart chakra is said to be "seat of the soul" as per Himalayan Tantric tradition. It is one of the most powerful centers of all, as it is linked to the lungs. We can picture the heart as a common ground for the wide collection of human emotional experiences. The heart as an organ has the ability to depict the greater aspects of life in a human being like spiritual compassion, unconditional love, and total faith. However, it can also depict the darker sides of our darker emotions, insecurity, disappointment, loneliness and helplessness. To activate your soul into the chakra of the heart, exercise with pranayama, focused meditation, and heartfelt prayer.

Vishuddhi (Throat Chakra) - The vishuddhi yoga center is linked with the element of ether. It is a powerful home for abilities like speech and hearing along with the endocrine glands that regulate your daily metabolism. On a spiritual level, this chakra is about enhancing your divine communication. To purify your throat chakra, we can work with chant, JalandharaBandha, with emphasis on various asanas like Plow, Camel, Shoulderstand, and Fish Posture.

Ajna (Third Eye Chakra) - The ajna yogic chakra also referred to as the "command center," is found below the eyebrow level with the mid-brain. It is a convergence point between two crucial energetic streams in the body, the ida, and pingalanadis, where the mind and the body fuse to one. When relaxed consciousness flows here, we have a feeling of purposture and feel more than just mortal. To isolate your mind to the chakra, we can practice alternate nostril breathing exercises (nadishodhana) and meditations focused on the chakra location.

Sahasrara(Crown Center) - This yogic chakra is associated with your alternate and much more expressive individual ego. It is everything that you hide in someone above your linear intellect and personal requirements, desires and emotionality. By purifying this chakra, we can set a gateway linear path to enlightenment. ⍰

Chapter 6 – Enhance Yoga With Meditation

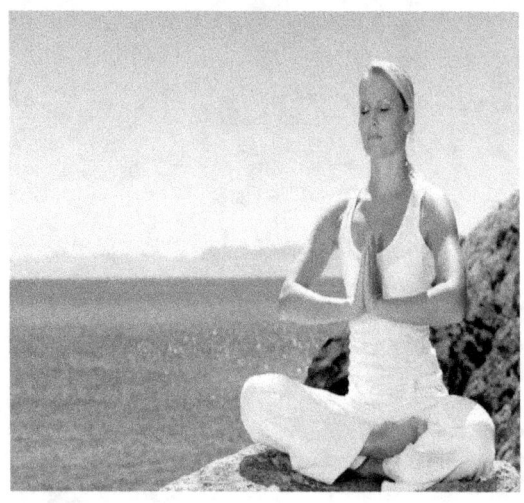

The advantages of meditation are known widely. It is a necessary form of exercise for the maintenance of mental health. A relaxed mind works with proper focus and clear thoughts and enhanced communication, springing skills and talents. Cognizant strength, healing, and the ability to associate with a greater and deeper form of energy, serenity, rejuvenation, and hard work are all natural consequences of regular meditation. Meditation is a yogic exercise

that gives you deep rest that is far from what you get when you sleep daily. Resting in meditation is more relaxing than the most comfortable sleep you ever could have. Meditation is when and where the mind is free from all forms of agitation. It is calm and peaceful and when in peace, meditation happens.
For inculcating the process of meditation, everyone has to go through few checkpoints before they jump into the main event unprepared. In a fast paced technologically challenging world where tension and stress levels peak with time, the mind is deeply affected which makes meditation a need rather than a luxury. It is a necessity, which one has to complete to be truly happy with inner peace all through the power of meditation.

Beginners must follow the below-listed tips in the field of yogic meditation:

Deep Outward Breathing - Yoga is not a physical entity. It is all about a simple process of uniting yourself – your soul and body together by using your breath, body, and the mind easily and effortlessly.

Following the guidance - It is recommended to initiate the process of learning the yoga practice under the able guidance of an experienced yoga teacher who can lead you to a path of righteousness with each technique. This would help you learn the concepts of yoga accurately and avoid physical strain. It is ideal to open yourself up to broaden and enhance your yoga experience.

Conscious and safe practicing - If you have a medical condition, informing your yoga instructor before commencing your training program is recommended. It will help the teacher regulate and improve your training without hurting you.

Simple attire - Comfortable clothing or clothing you feel relaxed in is ideal for a yoga class or even while practicing yoga at home as it does not block your progress. Avoid wearing belts or excessive jewelry as it could obstruct your yoga practice.

Early rising - Although it is advised to practice yoga postures early in the morning, practically it is not possible every day. Importantly, practicing at any time of the day as per convenience is much more beneficial.

Light eating - Yoga on an empty stomach or at least 2-3 hours after your last meal is more effective and advised. Also, drink enough fluids to properly hydrate your body and eat healthy foods.

Warming up - Casual warm up exercises will loosen up the body early to prepare you for the strenuous yoga postures to come.

Relaxed and happy mind - See the difference in yourself when you keep a gentle smile. Your body and mind will feel relaxed and help you benefit from the yoga postures.

Steady practicing - Practice as much as you comfortably can and try to just stretch a bit more regularly to enhance body flexibility. Use your breath as a reference point, when it is lighter, the muscles begin to relax, but when it is uneven and irregularly paced, it means you are tense.

Building stamina gradually - Different people are at different levels of expertise, and a common line cannot be drawn. The muscles get sore during the first few days of practice, and that has nothing to do with your stamina levels. Avoid comparing yourself to other people like the students in the yoga class. Every body type is unique and capable. Inform your instructor immediately in case you are feeling persisting pain.

Energy restoration - As you complete yoga posture practice, don't be in a great hurry. It is extremely good to lie down in Yoga Nidra for a couple of minutes, cooling the body just like warm up. Yoga Nidra is also advantageous in enhanced relaxation of the mind and body after the meditation.

Follow Some Rules Before Meditating For Better Results.

Before Meditation

Take a relaxed posture for meditation as it is extremely important for the mind. If you have extra five minutes, you would want to stretch your muscles through a quick warm-up. This can be followed by a relevant yoga asanas or a few sets of SuryanamaskarKriya.

It is advised to cleanse yourself by taking a shower and wear a fresh pair of clothes to begin your session of meditation.

Empty stomach meditation is always preferred. Eating a meal might block the efficiency of your meditation as your body and mind aren't relaxed but are in a continuous state of work.

At the time of Meditation

If the outer world is all about hard work and precipitation, your inner soul wants you to put in the least efforts and work efficiently. Meditation is hence a seamless experience.

There are three golden rules to be followed by those who meditate -

I Do Nothing: There is no physical manifestation of Yoga. All you can do is breathe.

I Am Nothing: An individual in a single life plays several roles. Carrying an identity messes your mind and doesn't allow it to rest. During meditation, we drop our diversities and focus on our common inner souls.

I Want Nothing: For the 20 minutes of meditation, you do not have any persistent desires.

Post Meditation

A few minutes of silence after a session is recommended for digestion of thoughts and processes. It is not recommended to rush to your computer and television as it can cook the brain up. Get onto your work gradually, building a momentum. The sudden jerk of activity could be tasking.

You will feel hungry after your meditation. Have something fresh once you finish your meditation to quench your hunger, similarly repeat the meal pattern for the evening meditation.